LOW RESIDUE DIET COOKBOOK: MEAL PREP FOR BEGINNERS

Low FODMAP Recipes to Combat IBS, Diverticulitis, Gastroparesis, Colitis, and Crohn's Disease Flare-Ups

Sarah Hayes, RD

Copyright Page

© 2024 Sarah Hayes, RD.

The recipes and information presented in this cookbook are intended for general informational purposes only. While the author and publisher have made every effort to ensure that the content is accurate and up-to-date, no guarantee is given regarding the completeness, reliability, or suitability of the information provided.

Contents

CHAPTER ONE: UNDERSTANDING LOW RESIDUE DIET

What is a Low Residue Diet?

A low residue diet excludes or limits foods that contribute to stool weight, such as high fiber foods, including whole grains, fruits with the peel, and vegetables.

Doctors who recommend this diet intend it to be both diagnostic and therapeutic for people who:

Are preparing for a colonoscopy

Have inflammatory bowel disease (IBD), such as Crohn's

Are preparing for or recovering from bowel surgery

Have infectious colitis

Have acute diverticulitis

The intention of a low residue diet is to help clear or heal the colon by allowing time for bowel rest.

Healthcare professionals often use the terms "low residue diet" and "low fiber diet" interchangeably.

However, a low residue diet also involves limiting dairy products. Dairy contains little fiber but contributes considerably to gut residue and fecal bulking.

How it works

A low residue diet limits dietary fiber to 10–15 grams per day.

The goal is to reduce bowel activity and promote intestinal healing by minimizing the intake of indigestible material.

These indigestible materials include:

Fiber

Fiber, also known as roughage or crude fiber, is a carbohydrate the body cannot break down into sugar molecules. It helps the body regulate sugar and hunger. There are two types of fiber:

Soluble fiber dissolves in water. It is found in foods such as oatmeal, nuts, lentils, chia seeds, apples, and blueberries. Soluble fiber can help lower glucose levels and lower blood cholesterol.

Insoluble fiber is found in whole grains, legumes, leafy greens, nuts, seeds, and fruit. Insoluble fiber is indigestible, so it helps food move through the digestive system, encouraging bowel regularity and preventing constipation.

Residue

"Residue" refers to food that is low in crude fiber but contributes to waste. Foods that contribute to residue that are low in fiber include:

meats

fats

dairy products

When is a Low Residue Diet Recommended?

A low residue diet aims to produce fewer and smaller bowel movements to help clear the intestinal tract.

However, low residue diets were removed from the American Academy of Nutrition and Dietetics Nutrition Care manual in 2012.

Healthcare professionals no longer recommend a low residue diet for Crohn's disease, ulcerative colitis, bowel resection, and ileostomy.

However, some medical professionals may still recommend low fiber therapy in the following cases:

IBD: Crohn's and ulcerative colitis

Doctors may prescribe a temporary low fiber or low residue diet to people experiencing an active IBD flare to ease symptoms such as:

rectal pain

diarrhea

cramping

bloating

gas

bleeding

Colonoscopy preparation

Endoscopists typically recommend a temporary low fiber diet to people 24 hours before a colonoscopy.

Some endoscopists might recommend a 3-day low fiber diet, but there is no evidence to support it improves colonoscopy results.

Bowel surgery

People preparing for colon surgery, such as an ileostomy, colostomy, or bowel resection, may need to follow a low residue or liquid-only diet before the procedure.

They may also have to follow this diet after surgery to help speed healing.

While there is little high quality evidence to support the effectiveness of a low residue diet for colon surgery preparation and healing, some healthcare professionals may still recommend it based on their clinical experience.

One 2014 study included 111 people undergoing colorectal surgery. Participants who followed a low residue diet instead of a liquid diet after colon surgery had a quicker return to typical bowel function and shorter hospital stays.

Diverticulitis and IBS

Healthcare professionals may recommend a temporary low residue or low fiber diet to people with diverticulitis experiencing flare-ups.

However, people with diverticulitis should eat a high fiber, low fat diet when they are not experiencing a period of inflammation.

Additionally, healthcare professionals may suggest a low residue diet to people with irritable bowel syndrome (IBS) to help ease discomfort. However, it is more common for doctors to recommend a low FODMAP diet.

Benefits of a Low Residue Diet

The low-residue diet has benefits for specific circumstances. The main health benefits of a low-residue diet relate to digestion. People with IBD can expect to experience the most benefits from this diet. This is not a diet that is designed for weight loss.

May help with IBD: A low-residue diet is specifically tailored to provide relief for patients with IBD. Adopting a diet low in fiber gives the digestive system, specifically the large intestine, an opportunity to rest. While the bowels are not required to break down high-fiber foods, healing can occur.

May reduce gas and bloating: The diet is beneficial for people who experience frequent bowel movements and have inflammation in their bowels, as it gives the large intestine a break. With fewer stools, people following a low-residue diet may experience relief from symptoms like diarrhea, bloating, gas, and cramping.

Can prep bowels before surgery or colonoscopy: A liquid-only diet is often recommended before bowel surgery or colonoscopy. This is known as bowel prep. Up to a week before your procedure, you may be asked to avoid high-fiber foods, so your bowels are as empty as possible. This will reduce the number of bowel movements you take leading up to the procedure. You may need to modify the diet to incorporate more liquids than solids as the procedure gets closer.

May act as a transition from liquids to solids: People who have followed a liquid-only diet may need a gradual return to foods containing fiber. Adopting a low-residue diet as part of that transition can help followers of a liquid diet return to their normal way of eating over time. Going from a liquid diet to a high-fiber diet could cause discomfort in the gastrointestinal tract, so slowly increasing the amount of fiber is recommended.

Cons of the Low-Residue Diet

A low-fiber diet is restrictive and can reduce the number of bowel movements that occur. For some people, a low-residue diet poses more risks than benefits, which is why it is only recommended for a short period of time and for certain circumstances.

Low in important fiber: Fiber is important for heart health and lowering the risk of chronic diseases, including cancer and diabetes.1

Fewer bowel movements: If you are experiencing diarrhea, fewer bowel movements can be a productive step towards regularity. If you have regular bowel movements, a low-residue diet can negatively impact your regularity. Digestion is a vital part of the body's natural system to remove waste that could otherwise build up in the body and cause damage.1

May cause nutrient deficiencies: When you consume refined grains, you are eliminating the part of the grain that contains nutrition. This could lead to deficiencies in vitamins and minerals. As well, avoiding the skins of fruit and vegetables means avoiding the most nutrient-dense parts.

May cause hunger: Without the bulk of fiber, you may feel hungry. Refined foods may cause your blood sugar to spike, leaving you hungry soon after. Higher fiber diets are associated with healthy body weight.2.

Recommended Timing

If you have digestive symptoms you're hoping to manage through diet, meal timing is important.

For example, you might find you feel best when you can sit down to three regular, balanced meals each day. Or, you might find having smaller meals more frequently, along with nutritious snacks, is better for your digestion.

Listen to your body; if you have a digestive disorder, what works best for you may depend on whether or not you're having symptoms.

Remember, too, that eating less fiber means you're likely to be hungry sooner because food is digested in the stomach faster. You might need to snack more frequently throughout the day. Increasing your fluid intake can also help.

Modifications

A low-fiber or low-residue diet can be difficult to navigate if you have diabetes. Many of the recommended foods (such as white bread) are simple carbohydrates, which will increase your blood sugar.

If you have diabetes and need to be on a low-residue diet, continue to pay attention to portion sizes and count carbohydrates for each meal and snack. When choosing low-residue foods, focus on approved veggies and lean protein.

Eating a well-balanced diet is especially important if you are pregnant or nursing. If you have a digestive disorder, pregnancy may exacerbate symptoms. Your healthcare provider might suggest you make some temporary changes to your low-residue diet or take supplements.

If you are on a low-residue diet while preparing for a colonoscopy, you will need to avoid red or purple foods and drinks (such as beets, purple sports drinks, or red gelatin). These foods can temporarily discolor the tissue of your colon, making it look like blood during the test.

CHAPTER TWO: FOODS TO INCLUDE AND AVOID ON A LOW RESIDUE DIET

What You Can Eat

The main foods to eat on a low-residue diet include those that are generally easy to digest. On this diet, you can expect to eat select fruits, vegetables, grains, dairy products, meat, oils, condiments, and drinks. Foods that are difficult to digest or high in fiber—whole grains, raw vegetables, beans, lentils, and more—are not permitted while following a low-residue diet.

It can be difficult to know what to eat on a low-residue diet since most food groups are allowed, but there are restrictions within each food group.

There are some patterns to help understand what is allowed on a low-residue diet.

What You Can Eat

Grains

Refined or enriched white breads and plain crackers, such as saltines or Melba toast (no seeds)

Cooked cereals, like farina, cream of wheat, and grits

Cold cereals, like puffed rice and corn flakes

White rice, noodles, and refined pasta

Fruits and Vegetables

The skin and seeds of many fruits and vegetables are full of fiber, so you need to peel them and avoid the seeds.

These vegetables are OK:

Well-cooked fresh vegetables or canned vegetables without seeds, like asparagus tips, beets, green beans, carrots, mushrooms, spinach, squash (no seeds), and pumpkin

Cooked potatoes without skin

Tomato sauce (no seeds)

Fruits on the good list include:

Ripe bananas

Soft cantaloupe

Honeydew

Canned or cooked fruits without seeds or skin, like applesauce or canned pears

Avocado

Milk and Dairy

They're OK in moderation. Milk has no fiber, but it may trigger symptoms like diarrhea and cramping if you're lactose intolerant. If you are (meaning you have trouble processing dairy foods), you could take lactase supplements or buy lactose-free products.

Meats

Animal products don't have fiber. You can eat beef, lamb, chicken, fish (no bones), and pork, as long as they're lean, tender, and soft. Eggs are OK, too.

Fats, Sauces, and Condiments

These are all on the diet:

Margarine, butter, and oils

Mayonnaise and ketchup

Sour cream

Smooth sauces and salad dressing

Soy sauce

Clear jelly, honey, and syrup

Sweets and Snacks

You can satisfy your sweet tooth on a low-residue diet. These desserts and snacks are OK to eat in moderation:

Plain cakes and cookies

Gelatin, plain puddings, custard, and sherbet

Ice cream and ice pops

Hard candy

Pretzels (not whole-grain varieties)

Vanilla wafers

Drinks

Safe beverages include:

Decaffeinated coffee, tea, and carbonated beverages (caffeine can upset your stomach)

Milk

Juices made without seeds or pulp, like apple, no-pulp orange, and cranberry

Strained vegetable juices

Foods to Avoid on a Low Residue Diet

What You Can't Eat

On this plan, you'll stay away from:

Coconut, seeds, and nuts, including those found in bread, cereal, desserts, and candy

Whole-grain products, including breads, cereals, crackers, pasta, rice, and kasha

Raw or dried fruits, like prunes, berries, raisins, figs, and pineapple

Most raw vegetables

Certain cooked vegetables, including peas, broccoli, winter squash, Brussels sprouts, cabbage, corn (and cornbread), onions, cauliflower, potatoes with skin, and baked beans

Beans, lentils, and tofu

Tough meats with gristle, and smoked or cured deli meats

Cheese with seeds, nuts, or fruit

Crunchy peanut butter, jam, marmalade, and preserves

Pickles, olives, relish, sauerkraut, and horseradish

Popcorn

Fruit juices with pulp or seeds, prune juice, and pear nectar

Fruit

Fruits like peaches, pumpkin, apricots, and bananas are fine as long as you remove pits, seeds, peels, and skins. Fruits with seeds not easily removed, like berries, are not recommended. Canned fruit and fruit cocktail cups may be OK, as long as they don't contain fruits on the avoid list (berries, for example). Avoid dried fruit, especially raisins, figs, dates, and prunes.

Most fruit juice is acceptable as long as you choose varieties without pulp. You will want to avoid high-fiber prune juice, however.

Vegetables

Peeled vegetables that are well-cooked (or canned) are approved, including carrots, beets, and green beans. Raw vegetables are typically too difficult to digest—particularly chewy and tough varieties like celery. You may choose to completely avoid leafy greens like lettuce, though they may be tolerable when cooked.

White potato can be eaten mashed or boiled without the skin. Avoid any pickled vegetables or sauerkraut.

Grains

Stick to bread and pasta made with refined carbohydrates. Choose white rice instead of brown rice, wild rice, or rice pilaf. Soda crackers and melba toast are approved.

Use white bread or sourdough bread for making toast and sandwiches instead of whole grain bread like whole wheat, pumpernickel, and rye. Avoid high-fiber snacks such as popcorn.

Try hot breakfast cereals like Farina instead of oatmeal. Grits and cream of wheat are other options. Cold cereal choices include puffed rice or cornflakes. Avoid bran and any cereals with nuts, seeds, berries, and/or chocolate.

Dairy

Limit milk products to no more than 2 cups per day. Low-lactose dairy options like cottage cheese may be tolerable. Yogurt can be part of your daily servings of dairy but choose plain flavors. Fats like butter and margarine are approved as tolerated.

Protein

Eggs can be soft-boiled or poached. Avoid nuts and seeds; nut butter is OK as long as you stick to creamy varieties.

Choose lean meat without gristle and cook until tender. Avoid frying meat or adding heavy spices or seasonings. Tofu is an approved protein source for meals and can also be used as a base for shakes and smoothies. Avoid beans and legumes including peas and lentils.

Beverages

Drink plenty of water. Carbonated beverages like seltzer are allowed, though they may increase symptoms of gas. Caffeine from coffee, tea, and soda are aggravating for some people with digestive disorders, though they are permitted on a low-residue diet.

Avoid all alcoholic beverages including wine, beer, and cocktails. If your healthcare provider suggests caloric or nutritional supplements (such as Boost or Ensure), you may want to look for options that do not contain dairy (or limit intake to no more than 2 cups if it's dairy-based).

Desserts

Plain cakes and cookies made with refined white flour and sugar are typically easy to digest. Sweets that contain chocolate, coconut, nuts, seeds, or dried fruit should be avoided. Gelatin and ice pops are especially helpful if you are on a clear liquid diet. Jelly, jam, and honey are approved as tolerated, given they don't contain seeds or pits.

CHAPTER THREE: TIPS FOR PREPARING THE LOW RESIDUE DIET

A low-residue diet is designed to provide temporary relief from digestive symptoms like stomach cramping, diarrhea, gas, and bloating. It is not intended to be a long-term lifestyle change.

If you have an inflammatory bowel disease (IBD), such as Crohn's disease or ulcerative colitis, your doctor may recommend a short-term low-residue diet to ease gastrointestinal symptoms like gas, bloating, diarrhea, and cramping.

A low-residue diet allows some nutrient-rich foods, but it is also restrictive and may make it difficult to meet your nutritional targets. This diet is not recommended long-term and should be followed under the guidance of a doctor or dietitian. Usually, followers of a low-residue diet can gradually return to their normal diet once their symptoms improve.

Many of the foods on a low-residue diet are low in fiber, which is an essential part of a healthy diet. While a low-fiber diet may provide relief from gastrointestinal symptoms, it is not sustainable long-term.

Sample Shopping List

Shopping for the low-residue diet is fairly easy. The work is in how you prep the foods you buy (by, for example, removing skins and cooking everything thoroughly). This is not a definitive shopping list and if following the diet, you may find other foods that work best for you.

Beef

Chicken

Canned cooked tomatoes

Fruit (bananas, grapes, canned fruit, applesauce)

Potatoes

Asparagus

Green beans

Dairy (milk, yogurt, cheese)

Smooth peanut butter

Pulp-free orange juice

CHAPTER FOUR: DELECTABLE RECIPE IDEAS AND SUGGESTIONS YOU MUST TRY

DELECTABLE BREAKFAST IDEAS

Crumpets

Ingredients

2½ tsp dried yeast

240ml warm milk

2 tbsp unsalted butter, melted

2tsp sea salt

2tsp caster sugar

470g plain flour

½ tsp baking powder dissolved in 60ml warm water

vegetable oil, to grease

butter or cheese, to serve

Instructions

STEP 1

Stir together the yeast and 240ml warm water in a bowl and leave to stand for 5-10 mins. Add the warm milk, butter, salt and sugar, then tip in the flour and stir until smooth. Leave to stand for 30 mins.

STEP 2

Dissolve the baking powder in a little water, then leave to rise for 20-30 mins.

STEP 3

Oil a heavy-based frying pan with a little vegetable oil and heat over medium-low heat. Lightly oil four 9cm crumpet rings. Spoon batter into the rings so it comes halfway up the sides. Reduce heat to low, cover with a lid, or an upturned deep frying pan to give the crumpets space to rise. Cook until the tops look dry, about 10-12 mins.

STEP 4

Flip them over and cook for 5 mins until golden and firm. Repeat with the remaining batter. Serve toasted with butter or topped with cheese, melted under the grill.

Cinnamon roll pancakes

Ingredients

145g self-raising flour

1 tsp baking powder

1 tbsp golden caster sugar

1 tsp cinnamon

2 eggs

40g butter, melted

140ml milk

3 tbsp light brown soft sugar

1 tbsp maple syrup, plus extra to serve (optional)

1 tbsp vegetable oil

6 tbsp toffee or caramel yogurt, to serve (optional)

Instructions

STEP 1

Weigh the flour in a large jug or bowl. Add the baking powder, caster sugar, ½ tsp cinnamon and a generous pinch of salt. Whisk to combine. Crack in the eggs, add ½ the butter and all the milk, then whisk to a smooth batter. Will keep in the fridge overnight.

STEP 2

Stir the rest of the cinnamon, the light brown sugar and the maple syrup into the remaining melted butter. Add 3 tbsp of the pancake mixture and mix. Transfer to a squeezy bottle fitted with a small nozzle or a piping bag.

STEP 3

When you're ready to cook, pour a little oil in your largest frying pan, and wipe out any excess with some kitchen paper. Keeping the pan over a low-medium heat, spoon 2-3 tbsp mounds into the pan for each pancake, leaving space for them to expand as they cook. You should get three or four in at a time. Use the cinnamon mixture in your bottle or piping bag to pipe swirls on top of each pancake. When the pancakes start to set around the edges and you see bubbles appear on top, carefully flip and cook for another 2-3 mins until golden and cooked through. Keep warm in a low oven while you continue cooking the rest of the batter.

STEP 4

Serve the pancakes with extra maple syrup, if you like.

Carrot & pecan muffins

Ingredients

2 x 400g can cannellini beans in water, drained

2 tsp ground cinnamon

100g porridge oats

4 large eggs

2 tbsp rapeseed oil

4 tbsp maple syrup

2 tsp vanilla extract

zest 1 large orange

170g carrot, coarsely grated

100g raisins

80g pecan halves, 12 reserved, the rest roughly chopped

2 tsp baking powder

Instructions

STEP 1

Heat oven to 180C/160C fan/gas 4 and line a 12-hole muffin tin with paper cases. Tip the beans into a bowl and add the cinnamon, oats, eggs, oil, maple syrup, vanilla extract and orange zest. Blitz with a hand blender until really smooth – the beans and oats should be ground down as much as possible.

STEP 2

Stir in the carrot, raisins, chopped pecans and baking powder, and mix well. Spoon into the muffin cases – use a large ice cream scoop if you have one, to get nice even muffins.

STEP 3

Top each muffin with a reserved pecan and bake for 20 mins until set and light brown. Cool on a wire rack. Will keep in the fridge for a few days, or freeze for 6 weeks; thaw at room temperature.

Poached Eggs

Ingredients

1 tbsp white wine vinegar

eggs, as many as you want to poach

Instructions

STEP 1

Fill a large saucepan with water and add the vinegar. As soon as the water starts to boil, turn the heat down to a simmer.

STEP 2

Crack the egg into a small bowl. For a perfect egg with no wispy white bits, crack into a fine strainer and allow the runnier egg white to drain off.

STEP 3

Stir the water to create a gentle whirlpool which will help the egg white wrap around the yolk. Then carefully slide the egg into the water making sure the heat is low enough not to throw the egg around - there should only be small bubbles rising.

STEP 4

Cook for 3-4 mins, until the white is cooked through.

STEP 5

Remove gently using a slotted spoon and blot any water from the base on a tea towel or kitchen paper. You can add more than one egg to the pan but make sure each one has enough room.

Microwave scrambled eggs

Ingredients

2 eggs

2 tbsp whole milk

toast, to serve

Instructions

STEP 1

Use a fork to beat together the eggs, milk and a pinch of salt in a microwave-safe jug. Cook in the microwave on High for 30 seconds, then beat again and return to the microwave for another 30 seconds.

STEP 2

Beat again, breaking up any lumps of egg. Microwave for another 15 seconds, then beat again; the eggs will be loose at this stage so serve them straightaway if this is how you like them. If you prefer your eggs a little firmer, microwave for

a further 15 seconds, beat, then serve.

Vegan French toast

Ingredients

3 tbsp maple syrup

150g blueberries

2 tbsp gram flour

2 tbsp ground almonds

2 tsp cinnamon

200ml oat milk or rice milk

1 tbsp golden caster sugar

1 tsp vanilla extract

6 slices of thick white bread

grapeseed oil, for frying

icing sugar, for dusting

Instructions

STEP 1

Gently heat the maple syrup and blueberries in a saucepan until the berries start to pop and release their juices, then set them to one side in the pan. Whisk the flour, almonds, cinnamon, milk and vanilla together in a shallow bowl.

STEP 2

Heat a little oil in a frying pan. Dip a slice of bread into the milk mixture, shake off any excess and fry the bread on both sides until it browns and crisps at the edges. Keep the slices warm in a low oven as you cook the rest. Serve with the blueberries spooned over and dust with icing sugar.

Seville orange marmalade

Ingredients

1.3kg Seville orange

2 lemons, juice only

2.6kg preserving or granulated sugar

Instructions

STEP 1

Put the whole oranges and lemon juice in a large preserving pan and cover with 2 litres/4 pints water - if it does not cover the fruit, use a smaller pan. If necessary weight the oranges with a heat-proof plate to keep them submerged. Bring to the boil, cover and simmer very gently for around 2 hours, or until the peel can be easily pierced with a fork.

STEP 2

Warm half the sugar in a very low oven. Pour off the cooking water from the oranges into a jug and tip the oranges into a bowl. Return cooking liquid to the pan. Allow oranges to cool until they are easy to handle, then cut in half. Scoop out all the pips and pith and add to the reserved orange liquid in the pan. Bring to the boil for 6 minutes, then strain this liquid through a sieve into a bowl and press the pulp through with a wooden spoon - it is high in pectin so gives marmalade a good set.

STEP 3

Pour half this liquid into a preserving pan. Cut the peel, with a sharp knife, into fine shreds. Add half the peel to the liquid in the preserving pan with the warm sugar. Stir over a low heat until all the sugar has dissolved, for about 10 minutes, then bring to the boil and bubble rapidly for 15- 25 minutes until setting point is reached.

STEP 4

Take pan off the heat and skim any scum from the surface. (To dissolve any excess scum, drop a small knob of butter on to the surface, and gently stir.) Leave the marmalade to stand in the pan for 20 minutes to cool a little and allow the peel to settle; then pot in sterilised jars, seal and label. Repeat from step 3 for second batch, warming the other half of the sugar first.

Kedgeree

Ingredients

50g butter

1 medium onion, finely chopped

3 cardamom pods split open

¼ tsp turmeric

1 small cinnamon stick

2 fresh bay leaves or 1 dried

450g basmati rice

1 litre/1¾ pints chicken stock or fish stock, ideally fresh

750g un-dyed smoked haddock fillet

3 eggs

3 tbsp chopped fresh parsley

1 lemon, cut into wedges, to garnish

Instructions

STEP 1

Melt 50g butter in a large saucepan (about 20cm across), add 1 finely chopped medium onion and cook gently over a medium heat for 5 minutes, until softened but not browned.

STEP 2

Stir in 3 split cardamom pods, ¼ tsp turmeric, 1 small cinnamon stick and 2 bay leaves, then cook for 1 minute.

STEP 3

Tip in 450g basmati rice and stir until it is all well coated in the spicy butter.

STEP 4

Pour in 1 litre chicken or fish stock, add ½ teaspoon salt and bring to the boil, stir once to release any rice from the bottom of the pan. Cover with a close-fitting lid, reduce the heat to low and leave to cook very gently for 12 minutes.

STEP 5

Meanwhile, bring some water to the boil in a large shallow pan. Add 750g un-dyed smoked haddock fillet and simmer for 4 minutes, until the fish is just cooked. Lift it out onto a plate and leave until cool enough to handle.

STEP 6

Hard-boil 3 eggs for 8 minutes.

STEP 7

Flake the fish, discarding any skin and bones. Drain the eggs, cool slightly, then peel and chop.

STEP 8

Uncover the rice and remove the bay leaves, cinnamon stick and cardamom pods if you wish to. Gently fork in the fish and the chopped eggs, cover again and return to the heat for 2-3 minutes, or until the fish has heated through.

STEP 9

Gently stir in almost all the 3 tbsp chopped fresh parsley, and season with a little salt and black pepper to taste. Serve scattered with the remaining parsley and garnished with 1 lemon, cut into wedges.

Vegan tomato & mushroom pancakes

Ingredients

140g white self-raising flour

1 tsp soya flour

400ml soya milk

vegetable oil, for frying

For the topping

2 tbsp vegetable oil

250g button mushrooms

250g cherry tomatoes, halved

2 tbsp soya cream or soya milk

large handful pine nuts

snipped chives, to serve

Instructions

STEP 1

Sift the flours and a pinch of salt into a blender. Add the soya milk and blend to make a smooth batter.

STEP 2

Heat a little oil in a medium non-stick frying pan until very hot. Pour about 3 tbsp of the batter into the pan and cook over a medium heat until bubbles appear on the surface of the pancake. Flip the pancake over with a palette knife and cook the other side until golden brown. Repeat with the remaining batter, keeping the cooked pancakes warm as you go. You will make about 8.

STEP 3

For the topping, heat the oil in a frying pan. Cook the mushrooms until tender, add the tomatoes and cook for a couple of mins. Pour in the soya cream or milk and pine nuts, then gently cook until combined. Divide the pancakes between 2 plates, then spoon over the tomatoes and mushrooms. Scatter with chives.

Dippy eggs with Marmite soldiers

Ingredients

2 eggs

4 slices wholemeal bread

a knob of butter

Marmite

mixed seeds

Instructions

STEP 1

Bring a pan of water to a simmer. Add 2 eggs, simmer for 2 mins if room temp, 3 mins if fridge-cold, then turn off heat. Cover the pan and leave for 2 mins more.

STEP 2

Meanwhile, toast 4 slices wholemeal bread and spread thinly with butter, then Marmite. To serve, cut into soldiers and dip into the egg, then a few mixed seeds.

Rye bread with almond butter & pink grapefruit segments

Ingredients

4 tbsp almond butter (make your own with the 'goes well with' recipe, right)

1 grapefruit (you will need about 100g flesh)

2 slices rye bread, toasted (optional)

Instructions

STEP 1

Toast your rye bread, if you like. Segment the grapefruit and spoon the fruit, along with any juice, into a small bowl.

STEP 2

Spread the almond butter onto the rye bread, and top with the grapefruit, drizzling any juice over the top.

Healthy egg & chips

Ingredients

500g potatoes, diced

2 shallots, sliced

1 tbsp olive oil

2 tsp dried crushed oregano or 1 tsp fresh leaves

200g small mushroom

4 eggs

Instructions

STEP 1

Heat oven to 200C/fan 180C/gas 6. Tip the potatoes and shallots into a large, non-stick roasting tin, drizzle with the oil, sprinkle over the oregano, then mix everything together well. Bake for 40-45 mins (or until starting to go brown), add the mushrooms, then cook for a further 10 mins until the potatoes are browned and tender.

STEP 2

Make four gaps in the vegetables and crack an egg into each space. Return to the oven for 3-4 mins or until the eggs are cooked to your liking.

Eggs benedict

Ingredients

3 tbsp white wine vinegar

4 eggs

2 toasting muffins

4 parma ham

For the hollandaise sauce

125g butter

2 egg yolks

½ tsp white wine vinegar or tarragon vinegar

squeeze of lemon juice

pinch of cayenne pepper

Instructions

To prepare:

STEP 1

Bring a deep saucepan of water to the boil (at least 2 litres) and add 3 tbsp white wine vinegar. Lower the heat down to a gentle simmer.

STEP 2

Break the eggs into four separate coffee cups or ramekins. Split the muffins, toast them for a few minutes either side and warm some plates.

To make the hollandaise:

STEP 1

Melt the butter in a saucepan and skim any white solids from the surface. Keep the butter warm.

STEP 2

Put the egg yolks, white wine or tarragon vinegar, a pinch of salt and a splash of ice-cold water in a metal or glass bowl that will fit over a small pan. Whisk for a few minutes, then put the bowl over a pan of barely simmering water and whisk continuously until pale and thick, about 3-5 mins.

STEP 3

Remove from the heat and slowly whisk in the melted butter bit by bit until it's all incorporated and you have a creamy hollandaise. (If it gets too thick, add a splash of water.) Season with a squeeze of lemon juice and a little cayenne pepper. Keep warm until needed.

To make the eggs benedict:

STEP 1

Swirl the simmering vinegared water briskly to form a vortex and slide in an egg. It will curl round and set to a neat round shape. Cook for 2-3 mins, then remove with a slotted spoon.

STEP 2

Repeat with the other eggs, one at a time, re-swirling the water as you slide in the eggs. Spread some sauce on each muffin, scrunch a slice of ham on top, then top with an egg. Spoon over the remaining hollandaise and serve at once.

Warming chocolate & banana porridge

Ingredients

120g rolled porridge oats

4 tsp cocoa powder

1 tsp vanilla extract

4 bananas, 2 chopped

2 x 150ml pots bio yogurt

milk, to serve (optional)

Instructions

STEP 1

Put the oats, cocoa and vanilla in a large bowl and pour over 800ml – 1 litre cold water (depending how thick you like your porridge). Cover the bowl and leave to soak overnight.

STEP 2

The next morning, tip the contents into a saucepan with the chopped banana. Cook over a medium heat for 15 mins, stirring frequently, until the oats are cooked.

STEP 3

Put half of the mixture in the fridge for the next day. Spoon the rest into two bowls, swirl in 1 pot yogurt and slice over a banana (save the other pot and banana for the next morning). Warm through with a splash of milk to reheat.

Poached eggs with smoked salmon and bubble & squeak

Ingredients

1 tbsp rapeseed oil

140g white cabbage, finely chopped

2 spring onions, finely sliced

300g whole new potato

1 tbsp snipped chives

2 medium eggs, at room temperature

75g smoked salmon

Instructions

STEP 1

Cook the potatoes in a pan of boiling water until tender, then drain.

STEP 2

Heat the oil in a non-stick frying pan or wok. Sweat the cabbage and the spring onions in the pan for a couple of mins. Meanwhile, chop and squash the potatoes roughly, then add to the pan along with the chives. Cook for 4-5 mins, flip it over (don't worry if it breaks) and cook for a further 4-5 mins.

STEP 3

Meanwhile, bring a small pan of water to a rolling boil, then reduce the heat so it is just simmering. Crack the eggs into the pan and simmer for about 3 mins until the whites are cooked and the yolk is just beginning to set. Remove with a slotted spoon and drain on kitchen paper.

STEP 4

To serve, divide the bubble & squeak between 2 plates, place the smoked salmon and poached eggs on top and grind over a little black pepper, to taste.

DELECTABLE LUNCH IDEAS

Flaked salmon salad with honey dressing

Ingredients

2 generous handfuls baby salad leaves, rocket or lamb's lettuce

140g sugar snap pea

1 avocado, stoned, peeled and diced

2 cooked salmon fillets (from Crispy Asian salmon, see 'goes well with'), flaked, skin removed

small handful coriander, finely chopped

For the dressing

½ tsp clear honey

1 tbsp boiling (or very hot) water

2 tsp cider vinegar

1 tsp tamari or soy sauce

1 tbsp mirin (use Sherry or sweet Marsala wine if you don't have mirin)

Instructions

STEP 1

For the dressing, put the honey and hot water in a jar, and shake vigorously to loosen the honey. Add the other dressing Ingredients and mix well.

STEP 2

Put the salad leaves, sugar snap peas and avocado in a large bowl or plastic container, and mix together. Scatter the salmon and the coriander on top. Serve directly from the bowl with the dressing on the side.

Spiced parsnip & cauliflower soup

Ingredients

1 tbsp olive oil

1 medium cauliflower, cut into florets

3 parsnips, chopped

2 onions, chopped

1 tbsp fennel seed

1 tsp coriander seed

½ tsp turmeric

3 garlic cloves, sliced

1-2 green chillies, deseeded and chopped

5cm piece ginger, sliced

zest and juice 1 lemon

1l vegetable stock

handful coriander, chopped

Instructions

STEP 1

Heat the oil in a large saucepan and add the vegetables. Cover partially and sweat slowly for 10-15 mins until soft but not brown. In a separate pan, dry-roast the spices with a pinch of salt for a few mins until fragrant. Grind with a pestle and mortar to a fine powder.

STEP 2

Add the garlic, chilli, ginger and spices to the vegetables, and cook for about 5 mins, stirring regularly. Add the lemon zest and juice. Pour in the stock, topping up if necessary to just cover the veg. Simmer for 25-30 mins until all the vegetables are tender.

STEP 3

Purée with a blender until smooth. Dilute the consistency with more water if needed, until you get a thick but easily pourable soup. Season generously, stir in the coriander and add more lemon juice to balance the taste. Eat straight away or chill in the fridge to reheat. This also freezes beautifully. Serve with crusty bread, if you like.

Spicy tuna & cottage cheese jacket

Ingredients

225g can tuna, drained

½ red chilli, chopped

1 spring onion, sliced

handful halved cherry tomatoes

½ small bunch coriander, chopped

1 medium-sized jacket potato

150g low-fat cottage cheese

Instructions

STEP 1

Preheat the oven to 180C/Gas 4/fan oven 160C. Prick the potato several times with a fork and put it straight onto a shelf in the hottest part of the oven. Bake for approximately 1 hour, or until it is soft inside.

STEP 2

Mix tuna with chilli, spring onion, cherry tomatoes and coriander. Split jacket potato and fill with the tuna mix and cottage cheese.

Goat's cheese, tomato & olive triangles

Ingredients

3 triangular bread thins

50g soft goat's cheese

2 x 5cm lengths of cucumber, thinly sliced lengthways

3 tomatoes, sliced

4 Kalamata olives, finely chopped

2 small handfuls rocket leaves

Instructions

STEP 1

Follow our triangular bread-thins recipe to make
your own.

STEP 2

Cut the bread thins in half, put cut-side up and
spread with the goat's cheese. Top with the
cucumber and tomato, then scatter over the olives
and top with the rocket. Eat straight away or pack
into lunchboxes for later.

Classic Swedish meatballs

Ingredients

400g lean pork mince

1 egg, beaten

1 small onion, finely chopped or grated

85g fresh white breadcrumbs

1 tbsp finely chopped dill, plus extra to serve

1tbsp each olive oil and butter

2 tbsp plain flour

400ml hot beef stock (from a cube is fine)

Instructions

STEP 1

In a bowl, mix the mince with the egg, onion, breadcrumbs, dill and seasoning. Form into small meatballs about the size of walnuts – you should get about 20.

STEP 2

Heat the olive oil in a large non-stick frying pan and brown the meatballs. You may have to do this in 2 batches. Remove from pan, melt the butter, then sprinkle over the flour and stir well. Cook for 2 mins, then slowly whisk in the stock. Keep whisking until it is a thick gravy, then return the meatballs to the pan and heat through. Sprinkle with dill and serve with cranberry jelly, greens and mash.

Parmesan pork with tomato & olive spaghetti

Ingredients

300g lean pork fillet, cut into 6 equal slices

3 tsp rapeseed oil

3 tsp finely chopped fresh sage

4 garlic cloves, finely grated

15g very finely grated parmesan

1 large carrot (215g), chopped

3 celery sticks (165g), chopped

6 Kalamata olives, thinly sliced

2 tbsp tomato purée

1 ½ tsp vegetable bouillon powder

150g wholemeal spaghetti

100g cherry tomatoes, halved

large handful chopped parsley (about 10g)

Instructions

STEP 1

Put the pork in a bowl with 1 tsp oil, 1 tsp sage, 1 garlic clove and lots of black pepper. Mix well, put on a tray and scatter with the cheese.

STEP 2

Heat the remaining 2 tsp oil in a pan and fry the carrot, celery and remaining garlic and sage for 5 mins, stirring frequently. Add the olives, tomato purée, bouillon and 200ml water, cover and cook for 5-8 mins or until the veg is tender.

STEP 3

Meanwhile, cook the spaghetti following pack instructions and heat the grill. Grill the pork for 6 mins, then leave to rest. Drain the spaghetti, reserving a little water, and toss into the veg with

the tomatoes and parsley. Add the water to loosen,
then serve with the pork.

Superhealthy salmon salad

Ingredients

100g couscous

1 tbsp olive oil

2 salmon fillets

200g sprouting broccoli, roughly shredded, larger
stalks removed

juice 1 lemon

seeds from half a pomegranate

small handful pumpkin seeds

2 handfuls watercress

olive oil and extra lemon wedges, to serve

Instructions

STEP 1

Heat water in a tier steamer. Season the couscous, then toss with 1 tsp oil. Pour boiling water over the couscous so it covers it by 1cm, then set aside. When the water in the steamer comes to the boil, tip the broccoli into the water, then lay the salmon in the tier above. Cook for 3 mins until the salmon is cooked and the broccoli tender. Drain the broccoli and run it under cold water to cool.

STEP 2

Mix together the remaining oil and lemon juice. Toss the broccoli, pomegranate seeds and pumpkin seeds through the couscous with the lemon dressing. At the last moment, roughly chop the watercress and toss through the couscous. Serve with the salmon, lemon wedges for squeezing over and extra olive oil for drizzling, if you like.

Hummus & avocado sandwich topper

Ingredients

2 big spoonfuls hummus

½ small avocado, diced

squeeze of lemon

some chopped red onion

coriander leaves

some halved cherry tomatoes

slice wholegrain seeded bread or rye, or wholegrain pitta, to serve

Instructions

STEP 1

Top bread or fill pitta with hummus, then add avocado with lemon, red onion, coriander and cherry tomatoes.

Barley couscous & prawn tabbouleh

Ingredients

125g barley couscous

zest 1 lemon, juice of 0.5

1 tbsp extra virgin rapeseed oil

½ small pack dill, finely chopped

good handful mint leaves, chopped

½ cucumber, chopped

2 nectarines, chopped

125g peeled prawns, or a handful of cashews or pecans for a vegetarian version.

Instructions

STEP 1

Tip the couscous into a bowl and pour over just enough boiling water to cover, following pack instructions. Leave for no more than 5 mins, drain thoroughly, then fluff up with a fork and tip into a bowl. Stir in the lemon zest and juice with the oil, dill and mint, then add the cucumber and nectarines.

STEP 2

Toss through the prawns or nuts and serve on plates or pack into lunch containers.

Chicken wrap with sticky sweet potato, salad leaves & tomatoes

Ingredients

100g cooked sweet potato (from Lemon & garlic roast chicken, see 'goes well with')

2 multigrain wraps

200g cooked chicken, shredded (from Lemon & garlic roast chicken, see 'goes well with')

small handful salad leaves

small handful baby plum or cherry tomatoes, halved

Instructions

STEP 1

Mash last night's sweet potato so that it's very smooth, then divide the mixture thinly and evenly between the wraps.

STEP 2

Divide the chicken, salad leaves and tomatoes between each wrap.

STEP 3

Fold the wrap and roll up, making sure that you contain the filling. Eat straight away or wrap in baking parchment and string (or foil) for later.

Healthy tuna pasta

Ingredients

150g wholemeal penne

1 large leek (200g), halved, and thinly sliced

1 tsp olive oil

160g cherry tomatoes, preferably on the vine

198g can sweetcorn, drained

75g ricotta

160g can tuna in spring water, drained

handful of basil, chopped, plus a few whole leaves
to serve

Instructions

STEP 1

Boil the penne with the leek in a large pan of salted
water following pack instructions, until al dente.

STEP 2

Meanwhile, heat the oil in a large pan over a
medium-high heat and fry the tomatoes for a few
minutes, until they start to burst and soften. Add
the sweetcorn and cook for 2-3 mins to heat
through. Drain the pasta and leeks, reserving a

little of the pasta water. Tip the drained pasta and leeks into the pan with the tomatoes, then toss through the ricotta and tuna.

STEP 3

Season with plenty of black pepper. If you want to loosen the consistency, stir in some of the reserved pasta water along with the chopped basil. Serve scattered with the whole basil leaves.

Wild salmon veggie bowl

Ingredients

2 carrots

1large courgette

2 cooked beetroot, diced

2 tbsp balsamic vinegar

⅓ small pack dill, chopped, plus some extra fronts (optional)

1small red onion, finely chopped

280g poached or canned wild salmon

2 tbsp capers in vinegar, rinsed

Instructions

STEP 1

Shred the carrots and courgette into long spaghetti strips with a julienne peeler or spiralizer, and pile onto two plates.

STEP 2

Stir the beetroot, balsamic vinegar, chopped dill and red onion together in a small bowl, then spoon on top of the veg. Flake over chunks of the salmon and scatter with the capers and extra dill, if you like.

Halloumi, carrot & orange salad

Ingredients

2 large oranges

1½ tbsp wholegrain mustard

1½ tsp honey

1 tbsp white wine vinegar

3 tbsp rapeseed or olive oil, plus extra for frying

2 large carrots, peeled

225g block halloumi, sliced

100g bag watercress or baby spinach

Instructions

STEP 1

Cut the peel and pith away from the oranges. Use a small serrated knife to segment the orange, catching any juices in a bowl, then squeeze any excess juice from the off-cut pith into the bowl as well. Add the mustard, honey, vinegar, oil and some seasoning to the bowl and mix well.

STEP 2

Using a vegetable peeler, peel carrot ribbons into the dressing bowl and toss gently. Heat a drizzle of oil in a frying pan and cook the halloumi for a few mins until golden on both sides. Toss the watercress through the dressed carrots. Arrange the watercress mixture on plates and top with the halloumi and oranges.

Vegan burritos

Ingredients

4 large or 8 small tortilla wraps

2 large handfuls spinach leaves, shredded

1 avocado, thinly sliced (optional)

hot sauce, to serve

For the chipotle black beans

1 tbsp oil

1 garlic clove, crushed

1 tbsp chipotle paste

400g can chopped tomatoes

400g black beans, drained

1 bunch coriander, chopped

For the lime and red onion rice

250g wholegrain rice, cooked and drained

1 lime, juiced

½ red onion, very finely chopped

50g hazelnuts, roughly chopped

Instructions

STEP 1

To make the beans, heat the oil in a pan and fry the garlic for a minute, then stir in the chipotle paste. Tip in the tomatoes, stir and bring to a simmer. Season with salt. Simmer until thick, add the beans and cook briefly (make sure any water gets cooked off), then stir in the coriander.

STEP 2

If you are using cold cooked rice, then warm it through, stir in the lime juice, red onion and nuts and season well.

STEP 3

Lay out the tortillas and sprinkle over some spinach, add some avocado slices and some rice, then top with the bean mix. Add a shake of hot sauce, if you like. Roll the bottom up, then fold the sides in to stop the filling falling out as you roll. Wrap tightly in foil, if you like, and cut in half.

DELECTABLE DINNER IDEAS

Vegan mac and cheese

Ingredients

160g raw cashews

200g carrots, peeled and cut into 1cm cubes

700g potatoes, peeled and cut into 1cm cubes

90ml olive oil

40g nutritional yeast

1 lemon, juice only

4 garlic cloves, peeled and roughly chopped

1 tbsp Dijon mustard

1 tbsp white wine vinegar

1 tsp cayenne pepper

400g macaroni

3 tbsp panko breadcrumbs

Instructions

STEP 1

The night before, soak the cashew nuts in water and leave overnight.

STEP 2

Heat the oven to 180C/160C fan/gas 4. Steam the carrots and potatoes together for 5 mins, until completely softened. Transfer to a food processor. Drain the cashews and add these with 60ml of the oil, then blitz to break down the nuts. Tip in the other Ingredients – apart from the macaroni, breadcrumbs and the remaining oil – then blitz again until the mixture is smooth and season well. Add a splash of water and just a drizzle of olive oil if it looks too stiff, then set aside.

STEP 3

Cook the macaroni in a large pan of salted water for 1 min less than packet instructions, drain then stir through the sauce. Transfer the mix to an ovenproof dish, stir the breadcrumbs with the remaining oil and some seasoning. Scatter over the top of the macaroni and bake for 20-25 mins until piping hot and crisp.

Chestnut, spinach & blue cheese en croûte

Ingredients

50g butter

500g pack leeks, thickly sliced

3 garlic cloves, thinly sliced

240g bag baby spinach

415g can chestnut purée

3 large eggs, plus 1 for glazing

½ nutmeg, finely grated

200g pack vacuum-packed whole cooked chestnuts, halved

85g fresh white breadcrumbs

220g pack blue Shropshire cheese, rind trimmed, diced

500g pack all-butter puff pastry

For the sauce

500ml vegetable stock

2 leeks, thinly sliced

1 tbsp cornflour

300ml pot double cream

Instructions

STEP 1

Melt the butter in a large frying pan. Add the leeks and garlic, stir well, cover and cook for 10 mins until the leeks are soft, stirring a few times to check that they don't catch. Tip into a large bowl. Put the spinach in the pan and allow it to wilt. Leave to cool and, when cold, squeeze out as much liquid from it as you possibly can.

STEP 2

Tip the chestnut purée into the bowl with the leeks and add the 3 eggs, the nutmeg, chestnuts, spinach, breadcrumbs, cheese and seasoning, and stir until well mixed. Chill for at least 1 hr until the mixture firms up.

STEP 3

Heat oven to 220C/200C fan/gas 7. On a lightly floured work surface, roll out the pastry to a rectangle large enough to completely enclose the filling. Carefully lift onto a large, long baking tray that has been lined with baking parchment, then brush round all the edges of the pastry with the remaining egg. Spoon the filling down the centre of the length of the pastry, leaving the ends clear. Tuck the ends over the filling, then firmly lift up the sides to wrap them round, trimming away any excess pastry as you go. Brush with more egg to glaze, then make a few holes in the top so steam can escape as it cooks. Bake for 40 mins until golden and the filling is firm. Remove from the oven, brush with more glaze and bake for 10 mins more.

STEP 4

To make the sauce, heat the stock in a medium pan, add the leeks, boil for 5 mins, then take off the heat and scoop out 2 tbsp of the leeks. Blitz the rest in the pan with the cornflour using a hand blender, then cook, stirring, until thickened. Pour in the cream and reserved leeks and warm through. Can be made 2 days ahead and chilled. Serve the pastry in thick slices with the sauce.

Molten cheese-stuffed burgers

Ingredients

1½ tbsp olive oil

1 onion, very finely chopped

70g smoked pancetta, finely chopped

1 garlic clove, crushed

4 thyme sprigs, leaves picked

500g lean beef mince (no more than 10% fat)

50g fresh breadcrumbs

1 egg yolk

60g mature cheddar, grated

60g grated mozzarella

For the herby burger sauce

120g mayonnaise

2½ tsp English mustard

½ small bunch of parsley, finely chopped

½ small bunch of basil

50g baby gherkins, finely chopped

To serve

4 seeded burger buns, split

2-3 Little Gem lettuces, leaves separated

2 ripe tomatoes, sliced

crispy fried onions

Instructions

STEP 1

Heat the oil in a frying pan over a medium heat
and fry the onion with a good pinch of salt for 15
mins until soft and translucent. Add the pancetta
and cook for 5 mins more, then add the garlic and
thyme, and cook for 2 mins. Remove from the heat
and leave to cool for 15 mins.

STEP 2

Tip the mince into a large bowl. Massage with
your hands for 5 mins to tenderise the meat, then

add the cooled onion mix, the breadcrumbs and egg yolk. Season generously. Divide evenly into four, weighing for accuracy, if you like. Mix the cheddar and mozzarella together. Form the beef portions into patties, patting each into a 10cm round. Divide the cheese mixture into four, and, in your hands, form each portion into a firm ball, then press into a roughly 4cm disc. Working one at a time, put a cheese disc into the centre of a beef patty, then bring the meat around the cheese to cover. Lightly pat with the palm of your hand to flatten slightly, then chill, covered, for at least 30 mins or up to 48 hrs.

STEP 3

Make the sauce by whizzing the mayonnaise, mustard and herbs together in a small food processor. Stir through the gherkins, then cover and chill until ready to use.

STEP 4

Light the barbecue. When the flames have died down, grill the burgers on each side for 4-5 mins until charred (if you don't have a barbecue, see tip, below). Wrap individually in foil and leave on the barbecue for 5-7 mins so the cheese centre melts.

STEP 5

Grill the buns, cut-side down, for 1-2 mins until toasted. Spread all the cut sides with the sauce, then fill with the beef patties, lettuce, tomatoes and crispy onions.

Apple, cheese & potato pie

Ingredients

30g salted butter

1 tbsp vegetable oil

2 large onions, halved and finely sliced

½ bunch of thyme, leaves picked

30g plain flour

500ml vegetable stock

1 tbsp wholegrain mustard

1 tbsp white wine vinegar

450g potatoes (we used Maris Piper), cut into 2-3cm chunks

3 apples, peeled, cored and chopped into 1-2cm chunks

150g mature cheddar, grated

For the pastry

300g plain flour, plus extra for dusting

70g cheddar, grated

150g cold butter, cut into cubes

1 egg, beaten

Instructions

STEP 1

First, make the pastry. Tip the flour, cheese and a pinch of salt into a large bowl and mix. Add the butter and rub it in using your fingertips until the mixture resembles breadcrumbs. Mix in 4-5 tbsp cold water, and bring together into a dough. Wrap and chill for 30 mins.

STEP 2

To make the filling, melt the butter in a medium saucepan over a medium heat, then add the oil and onions and cook for 10-15 mins until caramelised. Add the thyme and fry for 1 min more. Tip in the flour, and stir to combine. Gradually stir in the stock, adding it in small amounts to prevent lumps forming. Bring to a simmer and cook for 10 mins, stirring occasionally. Stir in the mustard and vinegar towards the end of the cooking time.

STEP 3

Meanwhile, put the potatoes in a large pan of cold water, bring to the boil and cook for 4-5 mins until just cooked and still holding their shape. Drain well, then stir into the sauce. Add the apples, cheddar and some seasoning, and stir again. Heat the oven to 200C/180C fan/gas 6.

STEP 4

Pour the filling into a 28cm oval baking dish (ours was 28 x 18.5 x 6.5cm). While it cools, roll out the pastry on a surface lightly dusted with flour to the thickness of a £1 coin. Cut into strips roughly 1cm wide. Lay half the strips across the dish horizontally, leaving gaps of a few millimetres in-between, then, one by one, weave in the remaining strips vertically, using an over and under technique, also spacing them apart by a few millimetres. Re-roll any trimmings and cut into flowers, leaves, or other shapes to decorate, if you like (see tip, below). Arrange any pastry shapes on top, then brush with the beaten egg.

STEP 5

Bake for 50 mins, keeping an eye on it – you may need to cover the top with foil if it's starting to brown too quickly. Leave to cool for at least 10 mins before serving.

Fish pie mac 'n' cheese

Ingredients

650ml milk

40g plain flour

40g butter

2 tsp Dijon mustard

150g mature cheddar, grated

180g frozen peas

handful of parsley, chopped

300g macaroni

300g fish pie mix (smoked fish, white fish and salmon)

green salad, to serve (optional)

Instructions

STEP 1

Pour the milk into a large pan and add the flour and butter. Set over a medium heat and whisk continuously until you have a smooth, thick white sauce. Remove from the heat, add the mustard, most of the cheese (save a handful for the top), peas and parsley.

STEP 2

Meanwhile, boil the pasta in a large pan of water following pack instructions until just cooked. Drain.

STEP 3

Heat the oven to 200C/180C fan/gas 6. Tip the pasta into the sauce and add half the fish, stir everything together then tip into a large baking dish. Top with the rest of the fish, pushing it into the pasta a little, then scatter with the remaining cheese. Bake for 30 mins until golden, then serve with salad, if you like. Can be chilled and eaten within three days or frozen for up to a month. Defrost in the fridge, then reheat in a microwave or oven until piping hot.

Macaroni cheese lasagne

Ingredients

2 tbsp olive oil

400g lean beef mince

50g smoked pancetta, chopped

½ onion, finely chopped

½ celery stick, finely chopped

½ carrot, finely chopped

1 garlic clove, crushed

150ml red wine

1 tbsp tomato purée

400g can chopped tomatoes

250ml beef stock

2 bay leaves

1 rosemary sprig

1 tsp sugar

400g macaroni

80g grated mozzarella

a few whole basil leaves, to serve (optional)

For the cheese sauce

50g butter

50g plain flour

2 tsp English mustard

800ml semi-skimmed milk

small grating of nutmeg

100g grated parmesan

100g mature cheddar, grated

Instructions

STEP 1

Heat half the oil in a large, heavy-based frying pan
or casserole dish over a medium-high heat, and fry

the mince and pancetta until golden. Transfer to a bowl using a slotted spoon and set aside.

STEP 2

Add the remaining oil to the pan and fry the onion, celery and carrot for 10 mins until just softened. Add the garlic and cook for 1 min more, then return the meat to the pan. Tip in the wine, bring to a simmer and cook until the mixture is reduced by half. Stir in the tomato purée, tomatoes, stock, bay, rosemary and sugar. Simmer, covered, for 30 mins, then remove the lid and simmer uncovered for another 10 mins until reduced. The ragu will keep in the freezer for up to two months. Leave to cool completely before freezing.

STEP 3

Meanwhile, make the cheese sauce. Melt the butter in a saucepan until foaming, then stir in the flour and cook for 2 mins. Stir in the mustard, then remove from the heat and gradually whisk in the milk in small additions. Return the pan to the heat and simmer for 5-6 mins, whisking continuously until thick and smooth. Add the nutmeg, parmesan and 80g of the cheddar, then season to taste.

STEP 4

Heat the oven to 200C/180C fan/gas 6, and cook the macaroni in a large pan of boiling water for 5 mins. Drain, then stir into the cheese sauce. Spread the ragu into the base of a large rectangular baking dish (ours was 28 x 22 x 5cm), then spoon over the mac 'n' cheese and gently spread out using the back of a spoon to cover the ragu. Top with the remaining cheddar and the mozzarella, and bake for 25-30 mins until golden and bubbling. Leave to rest for 5 mins, then scatter over a few basil leaves to serve, if you like.

Blue cheese gnocchi

Ingredients

2 x 400g packs fresh gnocchi

1 tbsp olive oil

knob of butter

1 large onion, roughly chopped

500g small Forestière or Portobello mushrooms, sliced

2 large garlic cloves, chopped

150g pack creamy blue cheese

small pack parsley, chopped

Instructions

STEP 1

Bring a large pan of water to the boil and cook the gnocchi following pack instructions. When they float to the top of the pan, they are ready. Drain and set aside.

STEP 2

Meanwhile, heat the oil and butter in a large lidded frying pan. Add the onion and mushrooms, cook for 1 min over a high heat, then turn down the heat to medium, put the lid on and cook for 5 mins, stirring a few times.

STEP 3

Remove the lid and add the garlic, cook for 1-2 mins, then stir the gnocchi into the pan. Scatter over blobs of cheese and the parsley.

Roasted fish Italian style

Ingredients

4 fillets of firm white fish

1 tbsp olive oil

500g cherry tomatoes

50g black olive

25g pine nut

large handful of fresh basil leaves

Instructions

STEP 1

Preheat the oven to fan 180C/ conventional 200C/gas 6. Take the fish fillets with the skin on, and season with salt and pepper. Heat the olive oil in a large pan and cook the fillets skin side down for 2-3 minutes until just crisp. Transfer to a large roasting tin, skin side down.

STEP 2

Cut the cherry tomatoes in half and scatter around the fillets. Cut the olives in half and scatter over the tomatoes, followed by the pine nuts. Season.

STEP 3

Put the tray in the oven and bake for 12-15 minutes, until the fish is tender. Remove from the oven and scatter the tomatoes with the basil leaves. Spoon onto four warm plates and top each with fish. Drizzle with a little extra virgin olive oil.

Fish pie tart with minted pea salad

Ingredients

500g pack shortcrust pastry (or make your own),
see tip, below left

1 egg yolk and 3 whole eggs

250g piece undyed sustainably sourced smoked
haddock

250g chunky unsmoked fish (we used sustainably
sourced cod)

200ml tub crème fraîche

½ pack chives, snipped

grating of fresh nutmeg

handful of cooked sustainably fished large
prawns, defrosted if frozen

25g sharp cheddar or similar cheese, grated

For the salad

250g frozen petits pois

2 x bags baby leaf salad with pea shoots in the mix

mint

2 shallots, finely chopped

½ tsp sugar

2 tbsp red wine vinegar

2 tbsp extra virgin olive oil

1 heaped tsp wholegrain mustard

Instructions

STEP 1

Roll the pastry until just thicker than a £1 coin, and large enough to line a 23cm fluted tart tin (about 4.5cm deep) with some excess. Line the tin with the pastry, trim off the excess with a roll of the rolling pin, then prick the base all over with a fork. Chill for 15 mins. Heat oven to 200C/180C fan/gas 6. Line the pastry with a sheet of over-hanging foil and press it into the corners of the tin. Fill with baking beans, lift onto a baking sheet and bake for 25 mins until the pastry feels firm. Remove the foil and beans, and bake for another 5 mins until biscuity. Beat the egg yolk and brush it all around the inside of the case. Bake for another 5 mins until golden and lacquered. Turn the oven down to 180C/160C fan/gas 4.

STEP 2

Meanwhile, prepare the fish and filling. Put the fish on a plate, cover with cling film and microwave on High for about 4 mins until the flesh flakes easily. Alternatively, steam or gently poach the fish, then drain well. Gently transfer the fish to a colander and drain until the pastry is ready. Beat the 3 eggs, crème fraîche, chives and nutmeg with seasoning.

STEP 3

Flake the fish into large pieces, discarding any skin and bones, pat dry with kitchen paper and put into the pastry case. Tuck in the prawns here and there.

Pour the filling over, scatter with the cheese, then bake for about 35 mins or until golden and set, with just a slight tremble in the middle of the tart.

STEP 4

For the salad, boil the peas for 1 min until just tender, then drain and cool in cold water. Drain well, put in a large bowl and top with the pea shoot salad and mint leaves; chill until needed. Mix the shallots with the sugar, vinegar, oil and mustard together to make a dressing. Season. Let the tart cool for a few mins before serving. When ready to serve, toss the salad dressing with the peas, pea shoots and mint.

Steamed fish & pak choi parcels

Ingredients

4 plaice, haddock or other MSC-certified white fish fillets

2 pak choi, thickly sliced

4 spring onions, shredded

1 red chilli, thinly sliced

3cm ginger, cut into matchsticks

2 tbsp reduced-salt soy sauce

juice 1 lime

1 tsp sesame oil

Instructions

STEP 1

Heat oven to 200C/180C fan/gas 6. Place each fillet in the centre of a large square of foil. Top with the pak choi, spring onions, chilli and ginger, then pull up the edges of the foil.

STEP 2

Mix together the soy sauce, lime juice and 1 tbsp of water then spoon a little over each fillet. Crimp the top of the foil to enclose the fish and make sure there are no gaps for the steam to escape.

STEP 3

Place the parcels on a baking sheet and bake for 10-15 mins until the fish is cooked through (this will depend on the thickness of your fish). Open up the parcels and drizzle over a few drops of sesame oil. Serve with rice.

Crispy sesame fish

Ingredients

100g breadcrumb or 2 slices white bread, blitzed into crumbs

1 tbsp sesame seeds

4 fillets skinless white fish, each weighing about 140g

2 tbsp plain yogurt

1 tbsp olive oil

Instructions

STEP 1

Heat oven to 220C/fan200C/gas 7. Tip crumbs into a bowl with half the sesame seeds. Brush fish fillets with yogurt and coat in the crumb mix. Lay on a baking tray and sprinkle over the remaining seeds. Drizzle with a little olive oil, then bake for 15-20 mins. Serve with oven-baked potato wedges.

Courgette & watercress salad with grilled fish & herbed aïoli

Ingredients

about 12 baby courgettes

olive oil

4 fillets white fish, skin on

juice 1/2 lemon

bunch mint, leaves picked

100g bag watercress (or use rocket)

For the herb aioli

2 egg yolks

1 tsp Dijon mustard

1 fat garlic clove

200ml mild olive oil

lemon juice, to taste

handful mixed soft herb (such as chives, parsley, mint, and dill) chopped, plus extra leaves to serve

Instructions

STEP 1

Heat a griddle pan. Rub courgettes in 1 tsp oil, season, then griddle until just soft. Set aside while you make the aïoli. Whizz egg yolks in a processor with the mustard, garlic and plenty of salt. Gradually add the oil until thick, then season with lemon juice. You can make this with a stick blender (see Know-how, above right). It will keep for a day in the fridge.

STEP 2

Season the fish. Heat a non-stick frying pan until very hot, add 1 tsp oil, then fry the fish, skin-side down, for 3 mins until crisp. Turn and fry the fish for just 30 secs-1 min more until it is cooked all the way through.

STEP 3

To serve, fold the herbs into the aïoli. Whisk 1 tbsp oil with the lemon juice, season, then use to very lightly dress the courgettes, mint and watercress. Pile onto plates, top with fish plus a dollop of aïoli, then scatter with herbs.

Fish cakes with vegetables

Ingredients

450g firm white-fleshed fish such as cod or hoki

1 egg white

2 tsp cornflour

1 spring onion, finely chopped

1cm/½in fresh ginger, peeled and finely chopped

200ml/7fl oz peanut or vegetable oil, for frying

For the vegetables

8 dried cloud ear mushrooms (worth looking for,
otherwise use dried shiitake)

1 tbsp finely chopped garlic

1cm/½in fresh ginger, peeled and finely sliced

1 small onion, cut into wedges

1 courgette, sliced into irregular chunks

half a cucumber, sliced into irregular chunks

1 onion squash, peeled and sliced into irregular chunks (optional)

3 tbsp chicken stock or water

For the sauce

3 tbsp oyster sauce

2 tsp light soy sauce

1 tsp golden caster sugar

1 tbsp rice wine

125ml chicken stock

1 tsp cornflour mixed with 1 tsp water

Instructions

STEP 1

Remove any skin from the fish fillets and then cut them into small pieces. Combine all the fish cake Ingredients, except for the oil, in a food processor with 1 tsp of salt and 2 tbsp of water and blend the mixture until it's a firm paste.

STEP 2

Form the paste into two cakes, about 1cm thick. Heat the oil in a wok or large frying pan and fry each cake for 3-4 minutes on each side until golden. Remove with a slotted spoon and leave to drain and cool on paper towels.

STEP 3

While the fish cakes are cooling, soak the mushrooms in warm water for about 20 minutes until soft. Rinse well in cold water, drain, and set aside. When the fish cakes are cool, slice them into finger thick bite-size pieces.

STEP 4

Tip the oil out of the wok, leaving about 11/2 tbsp. Reheat the wok over a medium heat, add the garlic, ginger and onion wedges and stir fry for 1 minute. Add the courgette, cucumber, squash (if using), mushrooms and chicken stock and stir fry for another 2 minutes. Mix the sauce Ingredients together then pour into the stir fry and continue to cook for another 2 minutes or until the vegetables are cooked. Return the fish cake pieces to the pan and mix gently to heat through. Serve at once with boiled rice.

Crisp-skin fish with asparagus

Ingredients

24 thin asparagus spears

2 ripe tomatoes

1 tbsp extra-virgin olive oil

4 salmon fillets, each about 140g/5oz

For the dressing

3 tbsp extra-virgin olive oil

1 tbsp small black olives

1 tbsp capers, rinsed

2 tbsp parsley leaves

Instructions

STEP 1

Snap the woody ends off the asparagus, and discard. Cut the tomatoes in half, spoon out and discard the seeds. Finely slice the tomato flesh, then cut into small dice. Set both asparagus and tomatoes aside.

STEP 2

Heat the 1 tbsp olive oil in a large frying pan. Season the fish with salt and pepper, and cook skin-side down over medium heat for about 3-4 minutes, gently pressing, until skin is crisped and golden. Turn and cook the other side for 3-4 minutes, depending on the thickness, until cooked.

STEP 3

Meanwhile, cook the asparagus in simmering salted water for 3-4 minutes. Drain well. For the dressing, gently warm the 3 tbsp olive oil in a small saucepan with the tomatoes, olives, capers and parsley leaves. Toss the asparagus in a little of the dressing. Arrange the asparagus on each of four warmed dinner plates, top with the fish, and spoon the warm tomato dressing around the fish.

DELECTABLE SIDE DISH IDEAS

Raggmunk

Ingredients

25g plain flour

75ml full-fat milk

1 medium egg

1 thyme sprig, leaves picked

175g firm potatoes, like Desirée, coarsely grated

1 large carrot, coarsely grated

1 tbsp vegetable oil

Instructions

STEP 1

In a large bowl, whisk the flour with half the milk to make a smooth, thick batter. Beat in the remaining milk, the egg, thyme and some seasoning. Tip in the potatoes and carrot and stir to coat with the batter.

STEP 2

You will need to fry the raggmunk in batches so heat the oven to its lowest setting to keep them warm. Heat the oil in a large frying pan and spoon in the mixture to make 2 x 7cm-wide fritters, flattening the mixture with the back of the spoon as you go. Fry until golden brown and crispy, about 2 mins each side. Keep warm and repeat with the remaining mixture.

Thai prawn & lychee salad

Ingredients

500g large cooked prawns

small pack mint, leaves picked

small pack coriander, leaves picked

20 lychees, peeled, halved and stoned

150g bag beansprouts

large handful roasted peanuts, roughly chopped

small handful crispy onions or fried garlic chips (optional)

For the dressing

1 red chilli (optional)

1 tbsp brown sugar

juice 2 limes

2 tsp fish sauce

Instructions

STEP 1

To make the dressing, bash the chilli (if using) using a pestle and mortar. Add the remaining Ingredients, mix together and taste for a good combination of sweet, sour, salty and hot, then set aside.

STEP 2

Combine the prawns, mint, coriander, lychees, beansprouts and half the peanuts with the dressing, and toss well. Pile onto a serving platter and scatter with the remaining peanuts and the garlic chips or crispy onions (if using). Put in the middle of the table and let everyone help themselves.

Cabbage steaks with apple, goat's cheese & pecans

Ingredients

1 firm, round cabbage

2 tbsp olive oil

1 tangy, red-skinned apple (we used Jazz)

1 tsp cider vinegar

about 300g goat's cheese (one with a rind from the cheese counter) cut into four thick slices (we used Soignon)

25g pecans, roughly broken

a few thyme sprigs, leaves only

good pinch of cayenne pepper or hot smoked paprika

1 tbsp maple syrup

Instructions

STEP 1

Heat oven to 200C/180C fan/gas 6. Cut 4 x 2cm slices from the middle of the cabbage, cutting through the central core and leaving it in. Brush all over with nearly all the oil, season well, and place on a baking tray. Roast for 20 mins, turning carefully using a fish slice or wide spatula halfway through cooking.

STEP 2

While you wait, thinly slice the apple, leaving the skin on, then toss in a bowl with the vinegar and what's left of the oil.

STEP 3

Layer the apples on top of the cabbage steaks, roast for 5 mins more, then top each steak with a wheel of cheese. Divide the nuts, thyme leaves and cayenne between each mound. Roast for a final 5 mins until the cheese is starting to melt and the pecans are toasted. Drizzle with the maple syrup and eat straight away.

Smashed celeriac

Ingredients

5 tbsp olive oil

4 garlic cloves, very finely sliced

2 red chillies, deseeded and finely chopped

few thyme sprigs

2 small or 1 large celeriac, peeled and cut into 1cm cubes

splash of white wine (optional)

Instructions

STEP 1

Heat the oil in a shallow pan and sizzle the garlic for 1 min until fragrant. Add the chilli, thyme and celeriac. Toss everything to coat in the oil, then season with salt.

STEP 2

Turn the heat down to a minimum, cover the pan and cook everything really gently for 40 mins or until soft enough to squash. Stir occasionally and add a splash of white wine or water if it starts to catch. When cooked, crush the celeriac lightly with a wooden spoon and serve. The celeriac may now be left to cool in the pan – reheat on the hob with a drizzle more oil.

Red cabbage with carrot & edamame beans

Ingredients

1 tbsp sesame oil

juice 3 lemons

2-3 tbsp sesame seeds

1 small red cabbage, quartered, cored and shredded (about 400g after shredding)

350g edamame beans, podded

350g carrot, coarsely grated

small pack coriander, leaves picked and chopped

Instructions

STEP 1

Mix the sesame oil, lemon juice and sesame seeds in a small bowl to make a dressing, then set aside. Boil a large saucepan of water, add the cabbage and simmer for 3 mins. Add the edamame beans and simmer for 1 min more. Drain the vegetables and run under cold water, then toss with the grated carrot, dressing and coriander.

Seared beef & papaya salad with tamarind soy dressing

Ingredients

300g sirloin beef steaks, fat removed

vegetable oil, for greasing

100g bag baby spinach leaves

2 ripe but firm papayas, peeled, deseeded and sliced

1 small pack coriander, leaves picked

1 small pack mint, leaves picked

½ large cucumber, sliced

4 spring onions, thinly sliced

1 red chilli, thinly sliced

3 tbsp crispy onion

For the dressing

2 tbsp tamarind purée

1 tsp grated garlic

juice 2 limes

3 tbsp soft brown sugar

1 ½ tbsp fish sauce

large pinch chilli flakes

Instructions

STEP 1

Season the steak well. Heat a lightly oiled griddle or frying pan. Sear the steaks for 2 mins each side, then remove and leave to rest for 5 mins. When rested, thinly slice.

STEP 2

Mix the dressing Ingredients together with 1 tbsp water until the sugar is dissolved. Arrange the spinach, beef, papaya, herbs, cucumber, spring onions and chilli on a platter. Pour the dressing over half the salad and sprinkle with the crispy onions. Serve the remaining dressing on the side or save for making another salad.

Buttered spinach with feta

Ingredients

400g baby leaf spinach

25g butter

1 tsp grated nutmeg

100g feta cheese (or vegetarian alternative), crumbled

Instructions

STEP 1

Wilt the spinach in the butter in a large saucepan over a medium heat for a few mins. Once wilted, grate in the nutmeg, stir in the feta and serve straight away.

New potatoes with cornichons & cream

Ingredients

500g new potato

500ml chicken stock

200ml double cream

2 tbsp cornichons, sliced

small handful parsley, finely chopped

Instructions

STEP 1

Cook the potatoes in boiling salted water until tender. Drain and allow to cool on a tray (not under running water.) When cool enough to handle, cut in half or quarters, depending on size.

STEP 2

In a saucepan, reduce the chicken stock by two-thirds. Pour in the double cream and reduce by half. Add the cornichons, parsley and some salt if needed, then add the potatoes. Coat the potatoes in the sauce and serve in a bowl.

Charred onion & tomato salad

Ingredients

2 bunches salad onions, trimmed

270g pack mixed small tomatoes, halved

50g bag watercress

For the dressing

1 salad onion, steeped in vinegar

2 tsp white wine vinegar

2 tbsp extra virgin olive oil

½ tsp wholegrain or Dijon mustard

good pinch of golden caster sugar

Instructions

STEP 1

Heat a non-stick frying pan until very hot. Cut the salad onions in half lengthways and cook for about 2½ mins each side, cut-side first, until charred and tender. Transfer to a plate while you prepare the rest of the salad.

STEP 2

Cook the tomatoes, cut-side down, for 30 secs-1 min until just softened and caramelised, then set aside with the onions.

STEP 3

To make the dressing, put all the Ingredients into a jar with some seasoning and shake well. When ready to serve, pile the watercress, onions and tomatoes onto a platter. Give the dressing a quick shake, then drizzle it all over the salad.

Warm potato & rollmop salad

Ingredients

250g Charlotte potato (or another waxy variety), quartered

1 small red onion, finely chopped

6 small gherkins, sliced

1 tbsp red wine vinegar

1 tsp wholegrain mustard

3 tbsp virtually fat-free fromage frais

4 Rollmops

Instructions

STEP 1

Cook the potatoes in boiling salted water for about 10 mins until tender, then drain and leave to cool a little.

STEP 2

Meanwhile, mix the onion, gherkins, vinegar, mustard and fromage frais together in a medium bowl. Add the potatoes, mix well, divide between two plates, then top with the fish. Great with a green salad on the side.

Lemony mushroom & herb rice

Ingredients

a mugful of American long grain rice

250g pack chestnut mushrooms

2 tbsp olive oil

2 large garlic cloves, finely chopped

5 tbsp chopped parsley

3 tbsp snipped chives

finely grated zest 1 lemon

Instructions

STEP 1

Fill a roomy saucepan with water, bring to the boil and tip in a heaped teaspoon of salt - the water will bubble furiously. Pour in the rice, stir once and return to the boil, then turn the heat down a little so that the water is boiling steadily, but not vigorously.

STEP 2

Boil uncovered, without stirring (this makes for sticky rice) for 10 minutes. Lift some out with a slotted spoon and nibble a grain or two. If they're too crunchy, cook for another minute and taste again. They should be tender but with a little bite. Drain the rice into a large sieve and rinse by pouring over a kettle of very hot water.

STEP 3

Meanwhile, chop the chestnut mushrooms into smallish chunks and fry in olive oil in a large frying pan over a high heat for 4 minutes until golden. Stir in garlic and fry for 1 minute.

STEP 4

Drain and rinse the rice and toss it into the mushrooms with the parsley, chives and lemon zest. Try a little and add salt if necessary. The zingy, fresh flavours go really well with grilled fish.

Perfect sautéed potatoes

Ingredients

1kg waxy potato, such as Maris Peer or Desirée

6-8 tbsp sunflower or olive oil

Instructions

STEP 1

Cut 1 kg waxy potatoes into chunks.

STEP 2

Bring a large pan of water to the boil, then cook the potatoes for 3 mins. Drain, shake out onto a kitchen paper-lined tray and leave to cool.

STEP 3

When ready to serve, heat 6-8 tbsp sunflower or olive oil in a large non-stick frying pan until you can feel a strong heat rising.

STEP 4

If your pan isn't large enough, fry the potatoes in two batches – rather than crowding them. Have kitchen paper ready to drain them on. Add the potatoes in a single layer, not too tightly packed.

STEP 5

Turn the heat to medium-high, so that the potatoes sizzle, but don't stir until they start to brown underneath.

STEP 6

Turn them all evenly 2 or 3 times until nicely browned all over – this can take about 7 mins.

STEP 7

Then lift out with a fish slice or large slotted spoon to drain on more kitchen paper. Sprinkle with sea salt.

Chicken & chorizo quesadilla

Ingredients

1 tsp olive oil

1 shallot, sliced

100g chorizo, diced

2 cooked chicken breasts, shredded

2 plum tomatoes, diced

320g pack soft tortillas

200g cheddar, grated

small bunch coriander, roughly chopped

Instructions

STEP 1

Heat the oil in a pan and cook the shallot and chorizo for 5 mins until the shallot is softened. Stir in the chicken and tomatoes. Remove from the heat.

STEP 2

Put half the tortillas onto baking sheets. Spread a little chicken mixture on each one. Scatter over the cheese and coriander. Sandwich with the remaining tortillas. You can make up to this point 2 hrs ahead.

STEP 3

Heat oven to 180C/fan 160C/gas 4. Cook the tortillas for 3 mins. Using a fish slice, turn each one over. Cook for 3 mins more until both sides are golden. Put on a board, slice into wedges and serve.

Scotch eggs

Ingredients

12 large eggs

800g good-quality Cumberland or Lincolnshire sausages, skinned

5 tbsp curly parsley, finely chopped

2 tsp Worcestershire sauce

2 tsp English mustard powder

2 tsp ground mace

12 rashers smoked streaky bacon

85g plain flour

140-200g/5-7oz dried breadcrumbs

about 1 litre/1¾ pints sunflower or vegetable oil, for frying

scraps of bread, for testing oil

Instructions

STEP 1

Put 9 eggs into a large saucepan. Cover with cold water and bring to the boil. Once boiling, set the timer for 5 mins. When 5 mins is up, quickly lift the eggs out with a slotted spoon and plunge into a big bowl of cold water.

STEP 2

Put the sausagemeat, parsley, Worcestershire sauce, mustard powder and mace into a bowl with plenty of seasoning. Break in 1 of the remaining eggs and mix everything together.

STEP 3

Crack remaining 2 eggs into a bowl, beat with a fork, then sieve onto a plate. Tip the flour onto another plate and season well. Finally, tip the breadcrumbs onto a third plate.

STEP 4

Bring a large saucepan of water to the boil. Drop in the bacon rashers, turn off the pan and fish out the bacon with a pair of tongs – it should be just cooked.

STEP 5

When the eggs are cool, tap lightly on a hard surface to crack the shell, then peel (Picture A). If you hold the eggs over the bowl of water as you peel, all the shell bits will collect in there and you can dip in the egg to wash off any fragments. Wrap a slice of bacon around the middle of each egg, overlapping, like a belt (Picture B).

STEP 6

Now finish coating the eggs. I set up the Ingredients along my bench like a conveyer belt: eggs, then flour, mince, beaten egg and finally breadcrumbs, plus a baking parchment-lined tray at the end to put the finished scotch eggs on.

STEP 7

Roll your bacon-wrapped eggs in the flour, shaking off excess. Take a good chunk of mince and pat out to thinly cover one hand. Sit the egg on the meat (Picture C), then mould over the mince to cover, squeezing and patting so it is an even thickness. You'll probably have a gap (depending on how big your hands are – just patch and pat with a bit more mince). Dip in the egg, shaking off the excess, then roll in the breadcrumbs to coat, and transfer to your tray. Repeat to cover all 9 eggs, then cover with cling film and chill for 4 hrs or overnight.

STEP 8

To cook, pour the oil in a large, deep saucepan to about 4cm deep. Heat until a small chunk of bread browns in about 1 min. carefully lower in a Scotch egg and fry for about 5 mins, turning gently, until evenly browned. Depending on your pan, you can probably do 2-3 at a time, but don't overcrowd. Lift out onto a kitchen paper-lined tray. (If you like your scotch eggs warm, pop them into a low oven while you fry the rest.) Keep an eye on the oil – if the scotch eggs start browning too quickly, the oil might be too hot and you risk the pork not being cooked before the Scotch egg is browned. If the oil gets too cool, the Scotch egg may overcook before it is browned. Enjoy warm or cold; best eaten within 24 hrs of frying.

Roasted sesame sweet potatoes & asparagus

Ingredients

750g sweet potato, peeled and cut into 2cm pieces

3 garlic cloves, sliced

thumb-sized piece ginger, peeled and sliced into matchsticks

½ tsp sesame oil

1 tsp Thai fish sauce

1 ½ tbsp reduced-salt soy sauce

1 bunch asparagus, ends trimmed, cut in half

1 tsp sesame seeds

Instructions

STEP 1

Heat oven to 200C/180C fan/gas 6. Put the potatoes in a large roasting tin and toss with the garlic, ginger, sesame oil, fish sauce and 1 tbsp soy sauce. Roast for 20 mins or until golden brown and tender.

STEP 2

Add the asparagus, 3 tbsp water and the remaining soy, and roast for 10 mins more. Sprinkle with the sesame seeds, then serve.

CHAPTER FIVE: TO SUM UP!

Low-Residue Diet Considerations

In addition to thinking about what you can and can't eat, there are a few other considerations to keep in mind.

General Nutrition

Following a restricted diet can make it difficult to consistently eat enough calories and get adequate nutrition. Your healthcare provider may suggest you take nutritional supplements to help prevent deficiencies in key vitamins and minerals.

Your healthcare provider may order blood tests to check your vitamin and electrolyte levels. If you have a deficiency, slight adjustments to your diet or taking supplements may be all that's needed to correct it.

If you need to be on a low-residue diet for a lengthy period, consider working with a registered dietitian to ensure you're eating as well-balanced a diet as possible.

Sustainability and Practicality

Many foods approved on a low-residue diet are plentiful at markets and grocery stores. Stock up on non-perishable items like boxed pasta and canned goods to have on hand if symptoms pop up suddenly.

If you are unable to prepare fruits and vegetables according to the diet (peeling and cooking, for instance) many varieties can be bought pre-cut, pre-cooked, or already peeled. You can also get pureed versions of many fruits and vegetables, which can be eaten as-is or added to smoothies, sauces, etc.

Flexibility

Whenever you're planning to change how you eat, you'll need to take the reality of your day-to-day schedule into account. Some diets can be challenging if you can't plan ahead, but many approved foods on a low-residue diet are readily available at the grocery store or can be easily packed as a snack.

Even dining out on a low-residue diet is possible as long as you ask about how food is prepared, what ingredients are included in the dish, and know when to ask for modifications (such as swapping white bread for wheat).

Dietary Restrictions

If you follow a special diet for another reason, such as a food allergy, carefully consider any diet that further restricts what you're allowed to eat.

For example, if you're on a gluten-free diet, you probably already avoid many of the whole grains and carbohydrates that are on the "avoid" food list.

However, you'll need to pay careful attention to the ingredients commonly used to make gluten-free bread, pasta, and cereals, including nuts, seeds, and brown rice.

If you follow a vegan or vegetarian diet, low-residue animal products, such as meat, eggs, and dairy, would be excluded. The typical alternative sources of protein for plant-based diets, like beans and legumes, are not recommended on a low-residue diet.